OVARIAN CANCER

EXPLORING ALL THE POSSIBLE MEANS FOR

HEALING OVARIAN CANCER

DR. J. WALLER

Contents

INTRODUCTION

One type of cancer that starts in the ovaries a woman's reproductive organs that produce hormones and eggs is called ovarian cancer. It is a dangerous illness that is frequently difficult to diagnose, going by the moniker "silent killer" since early signs might not be evident. Although it can strike women at any age, postmenopausal women are more likely to be diagnosed with this kind of cancer.

Genetic mutations, age, and a family history of specific cancers are risk factors. When symptoms do occur, they may include bloating, altered bowel habits, and stomach pain.

Tests for imaging, blood, and pelvic health are all part of the diagnosis. Chemotherapy, radiation therapy, and surgery are among the available treatment options. The prognosis is contingent upon the stage of diagnosis, with early identification leading to markedly better results.

Risk-reducing operations and specific lifestyle decisions are examples of prevention measures. The goal of ongoing research is to improve knowledge and management of ovarian cancer. Regular medical check-ups and increased awareness are essential for the early discovery and successful treatment of this illness.

CHAPTER ONE

What is meant by "ovarian cancer"?

One kind of cancer that starts in the ovaries, which are a component of the female reproductive system, is called ovarian cancer. The ovaries, which are found on either side of the uterus, are responsible for producing progesterone and estrogen as well as eggs (ova). Tumors are created when aberrant cells in the ovaries proliferate and divide uncontrolled, leading to ovarian cancer.

Ovarian cancer comes in different forms, with epithelial ovarian cancer being the most prevalent. Additional varieties comprise stromal tumors, which originate from the hormone-producing ovarian tissue, and germ cell tumors, which originate from the cells responsible for egg production.

Because there are rarely any obvious symptoms in the early stages of the disease, ovarian cancer is frequently difficult to diagnose. It is usually discovered at a later stage as a result. Chemotherapy, radiation therapy, and surgery are possible forms of treatment. The stage at diagnosis and the efficacy of the selected treatment are two examples of the variables that affect the prognosis. Increased knowledge of risk factors and routine medical checkups are crucial for early detection and better results.

Understanding and early detection of ovarian cancer is crucial.

Comprehending and identifying ovarian cancer at an early stage is crucial for multiple reasons, since a timely diagnosis greatly influences the prognosis and treatment results. The following are some major points that emphasize how crucial early detection is:

1. The Quiet Character of Ovarian Cancer:

Ovarian cancer is sometimes referred to as the "silent killer" as, in its early stages, it may not exhibit any signs.

Delays in diagnosis can occur from modest symptoms or symptoms that are incorrectly linked to other illnesses.

2. Diagnosed at an advanced stage:

Treatment for ovarian cancer is more difficult because it is often discovered at an advanced stage.

A greater incidence of metastasis the spread of the cancer to other organs and a decreased likelihood of total surgical tumor excision are linked to advanced-stage cancer.

3. Better Results from the Treatment:

Targeted medicines and surgical procedures are among the more successful treatment options that are made possible by early identification.

When ovarian cancer is isolated or detected early in its progression, treatment success is frequently higher.

4. Increased Success Rates:

Early detection of ovarian cancer is associated with much greater survival rates.

The prognosis for ovarian cancer in its early stages is better generally, and therapeutic success is more likely.

5. Decreased Intensity of Treatment:

Less aggressive treatment options may be made possible by early discovery, reducing the need for major surgery or intensive chemotherapy.

6. Maintaining Fertility:

Conservative surgical methods may be able to preserve fertility in certain patients of early-stage ovarian cancer.

It might be especially crucial to preserve fertility options for younger women with ovarian cancer diagnoses.

7. Life Quality:

For those with ovarian cancer, early identification improves their quality of life.

Early commencement of the right medication can help control symptoms and lessen the disease's impact on day-to-day functioning.

8. Strategies for Reducing Risk:

Those who are at high risk, such as those with a genetic predisposition or a family history, can take advantage of early detection to think about risk-reducing measures.

In high-risk groups, healthcare clinicians may propose risk-reducing operations or preventive interventions.

9. Developments in Customized Health Care:

Targeted therapy and tailored medicine based on the unique features of the tumor become possible with early diagnosis.

Treatment alternatives with fewer side effects and more efficacy could come from targeted therapies.

10. Emotional and Psychological Health:

Early detection can help people deal more easily with their treatment journey by reducing the worry that comes with receiving a late-stage cancer diagnosis.

Early diagnosis and understanding of the illness gives patients and their families more time to make educated decisions about supportive care and treatment.

Ovarian cancer is a stealthy disease, which makes early identification difficult. To mitigate this, knowing your risk factors, getting frequent checkups, and reporting any worrisome symptoms right away are essential. The pro-active pursuit of healthcare and raising public knowledge are important steps in improving the prognosis of ovarian cancer patients.

Ovarian Cancer Types

Because diverse cell types within the ovaries give rise to different subtypes of the illness, ovarian cancer is a heterogeneous condition. Stromal tumors, germ cell tumors, and epithelial ovarian cancer are the three primary forms of ovarian cancer.

1. Ovarian epithelial cancer:

The most prevalent kind, which comes from the cells covering the ovary's surface.

Subcategories:

The most common subtype of serous carcinoma is identified by cells that resemble the lining of the fallopian tubes.

Mucinous Carcinoma: Contains cells that secrete the sticky material mucin. Compared to serous carcinoma, it is less frequent.

Endometrioid Carcinoma: Often connected to endometriosis, this cancer resembles uterine lining cells.

Composed of clear cells, clear cell carcinoma is frequently resistant to conventional chemotherapy.

2. Stromal Growths:

Form in the stroma, the ovarian tissue responsible for producing hormones.

Subcategories:

Granulosa cell tumors: Usually produce estrogen and originate from the cells in the ovaries that nourish the eggs.

Sertoli-Leydig Cell Tumors: Infrequent tumors with androgen hormone-producing capabilities.

3. Tumors of the germ cells:

Description: Derived from germ cells, which are the cells that generate eggs.

Subcategories:

Dysgerminoma: A prevalent form that is frequently observed in younger women.

Endodermal Sinus Tumor: Mostly affects young women and children. Also known as Folk Sac Tumor.

Teratoma: Consists of a variety of tissues and cell types.

Choriocarcinoma: Similar to placental tissue, it is uncommon and aggressive.

4. Combination Stromal and Epithelial Tumors:

Combination tumors: those with both stromal and epithelial components.

5. Primary Cancer of the Peritoneum:

Description: Occurs in the peritoneum, the lining of the abdominal cavity, and is similar to epithelial ovarian cancer.

6. Cancer of the Fallopian Tube:

Description: Although closely linked to ovarian cancer, this cancer starts in the fallopian tubes.

Associated Risk: There may be a higher risk for women who carry specific genetic mutations, like BRCA mutations.

Determining the best course of treatment requires an understanding of the particular kind and subtype of ovarian cancer. The majority of occurrences of ovarian cancer are of the epithelial subtype, which is frequently the target of clinical research and treatment plans. Although they are less frequent, stromal and germ cell cancers need specific treatment methods because of their distinct features.

It is noteworthy that ovarian cancer is a complex disease since individual tumors within each subtype may exhibit unique characteristics and genetic alterations. Targeted treatments and customized treatment regimens are developing along with research, providing promise for better results for those suffering from ovarian cancer.

Hazard Contributors

The chance of having ovarian cancer can be influenced by various factors. It is important to remember that the presence of one or more risk factors does not ensure the development of ovarian cancer, and many women who receive an ovarian cancer diagnosis do not have any known risk factors. On the other hand, some women who have risk factors might not ever have the illness.

CHAPTER TWO

The following are typical risk factors for ovarian cancer:

1. Age:

Older women are more likely to get ovarian cancer.

As one ages, the risk rises, especially after menopause.

2. Family Background:

Women are more vulnerable if they have a first-degree relative (mother, sister, or daughter) who has experienced ovarian cancer.

An increased risk may also result from a family history of endometrial, colorectal, or breast cancer.

3. Hereditary Mutations in Genes:

Mutations in the BRCA1 or BRCA2 genes: Hereditary mutations in these genes greatly raise the risk of ovarian cancer.

An elevated risk of ovarian and other malignancies has been linked to Lynch syndrome, also known as hereditary nonpolyposis colorectal cancer, or HNPCC.

4. Individual Cancer History:

A history of uterine, colorectal, or breast cancer diagnosis may marginally raise the risk.

5. Menopause age:

Women who experience menopause after turning 50 might be at marginally increased risk.

6. Reproductive and Childbearing Factors:

Nulliparity: There is an increased risk for women who have never given birth.

Late Childbearing: The risk may rise if a person conceives their first full-term pregnancy after the age of 35.

Certain research points to a potential correlation between infertility and fertility treatments.

7. Endometriosis:

An elevated risk may apply to women who have endometriosis, a disorder in which tissue resembling the lining of the uterus grows outside the uterus.

8. Treatment with Hormone Replacement (HRT):

Progesterone-free estrogen-only hormone replacement therapy used over an extended period of time may marginally raise the risk.

9. Overweight:

There is evidence linking obesity to a higher risk of ovarian cancer.

10. Use of Talcum Powder:

Although the evidence is inconclusive, some studies have revealed a possible link between the usage of talcum powder in the vaginal area and an increased risk of ovarian cancer.

11. ethnicity

BRCA1 and BRCA2 mutations may be more common in Ashkenazi Jewish women, which raises the risk.

12. Individual Elements:

Smoking and a few other lifestyle choices may slightly increase the risk of ovarian cancer.

13. Late Menopause and Early Menstruation:

There may be a minor increase in risk if menstruation begins before the age of 12 or if menopause occurs after the age of 50.

It's critical to go through personal risk factors with medical professionals and have routine exams in order to detect problems early. It may be recommended that women who have a significant family history or who have known genetic mutations receive genetic counseling and testing. In addition, high-risk patients may be evaluated for preventive procedures such risk-reducing surgeries and the use of oral contraceptives. Ovarian cancer prevention and early detection measures require regular gynecological exams and knowledge of possible signs.

Symptoms and Indications

Ovarian cancer is frequently referred to as the "silent killer" since, in its early stages, it may not exhibit any signs. When symptoms do appear, they are frequently vague and might be mistaken for indications of other disorders. It's critical to recognize any possible symptoms and indicators, particularly if they intensify or persist. These are typical ovarian cancer symptoms and signs:

1. Pelvic or abdominal pain:

continuous pain, pressure, or discomfort in the pelvis or abdomen.

The discomfort could be nebulous and sporadic.

2. Bloating:

stomach fullness or bloating that lasts a long time.

The abdomen could seem enlarged.

3. Trouble Eating or Feeling Satisfied Fast:

Changes in appetite, feeling full after eating a small quantity, or difficulties eating.

4. Urine Frequency or Urgency:

a greater need to urinate or more frequent trips to the bathroom.

may be accompanied with a sensation that the bladder has not been completely emptied.

5. alterations in bowel habits

alterations in bowel habits, including diarrhea or constipation.

persistent, unexplained alterations in bowel habits.

6. Unexpected Loss of Weight:

unintentional weight loss without nutrition or exercise modifications.

7. Weary:

chronic exhaustion or lack vitality.

8. Back Aches:

Pain in the lower back that doesn't improve with typical therapy.

9. Changes in Menstruation:

Menstrual cycle abnormalities or bleeding after menopause.

10. Pain During Sexual Activity:

Sensation or pain during a sexual encounter.

11. Indigestion-Related Symptoms:

problems related to the digestive system, such as heartburn, nausea, or indigestion.

12. Breathiness Shortness:

respiratory difficulties or shortness of breath.

It's crucial to remember that these symptoms are not always indicative of ovarian cancer; in fact, they might be brought on by a number of different illnesses. But it's important to see a doctor for additional assessment if these symptoms are brand-new, bothersome, and regular. Since ovarian cancer is frequently discovered at an advanced stage, prompt medical attention and symptom awareness are essential for early detection and better results.

Women who have known genetic abnormalities (such BRCA1 or BRCA2) or a family history of ovarian or breast cancer may also be at higher risk. As such, they should talk to their healthcare professionals about risk-reducing measures and surveillance. Proactive management and early detection of symptoms require regular gynecological checkups and open communication.

Identification

A mix of clinical assessments, imaging tests, and, in certain situations, surgical techniques are used to diagnose ovarian cancer. Ovarian cancer diagnosis might be difficult because of the lack of identifiable symptoms and the difficulty of early detection. Key steps in the diagnostic process are as follows:

1. Clinical Assessment:

Medical History: The healthcare professional gets details regarding the patient's symptoms, risk factors, and family medical history.

Physical Examination: The size, shape, and health of the ovaries are evaluated during a pelvic exam. Nevertheless, routine pelvic exams may miss early-stage ovarian cancer.

2. Imaging Research:

Transvaginal Ultrasound: Sound waves are used in this imaging procedure to produce finely detailed images of the ovaries and surrounding structures. It might be useful in locating ovarian anomalies or masses.

Pelvic magnetic resonance imaging (MRI or CT scan): These diagnostic tests offer more precise details regarding the location, size, and probable metastasis of ovarian cancers to other organs.

3. Blood Examinations:

CA-125 Blood Test: Some women with ovarian cancer may have increased levels of this tumor marker in their blood. Elevated CA-125 levels, however, are not always indicative of ovarian cancer; they can also occur in non-cancerous situations.

4. autopsy

Surgical Biopsy: Frequently the most conclusive diagnostic technique, a biopsy is the removal of tissue for microscopic inspection. Surgery may be used to do this, and the kind of biopsy used will depend on the features of the ovarian mass.

Fine Needle Aspiration (FNA): A little sample of ovarian tissue is taken for analysis using a thin needle.

Core Biopsy: To take a core tissue sample, a bigger, specialized needle is needed.

5. Laparotomy or laparoscopy for exploratory surgery:

A laparotomy is a surgical operation in which a wider incision is made in order to check the ovaries, explore the abdominal cavity, and obtain tissue samples.

Laparoscopy: A minimally invasive procedure to view the ovaries and adjacent structures through the use of a thin, illuminated tube equipped with a camera. It can be applied to staging and diagnosis.

6. Setting:

Staging Surgery: To ascertain the full extent of the disease, staging surgery is frequently carried out if ovarian cancer is established. Prognostic information and treatment decisions are guided by staging.

Biopsy of Other Organs: Biopsies of tissues, lymph nodes, and other organs may be carried out during staging surgery in order to gauge the extent of cancerous growth.

7. Genetic Examination:

BRCA1 and BRCA2 Testing: To find mutations in the BRCA1 and BRCA2 genes, genetic testing may be advised, particularly if there is a family history of ovarian or breast cancer.

8. Pathology Examination:

Pathological Analysis: A pathologist examines tissue samples taken during biopsy or surgical operations in order to identify the type of cancer and evaluate its characteristics.

Because ovarian cancer lacks identifiable symptoms and is frequently discovered at an advanced stage, early diagnosis is difficult. A proper diagnosis requires prompt medical consultation, in-depth clinical assessments, and pertinent imaging studies. Following a diagnosis, treatment choices are guided by a multidisciplinary team's holistic approach, taking into account the unique features of the ovarian cancer. For continuous care, regular monitoring and follow-up are crucial.

Stage and Outlook

grasp and treating ovarian cancer requires a grasp of its staging and prognosis. The FIGO (International Federation of Gynecology and Obstetrics) staging system is applied to ovarian cancer. There are four stages: I, when it is limited to the ovaries, and IV, where it has spread to other organs. Numerous factors, such as the patient's general health, the tumor's grade, and the stage of diagnosis, affect the prognosis.

The prognosis for ovarian cancer is often better for early-stage cases (stages I and II) than for later cases (stages III and IV). While advanced stages may have a reduced survival probability, stage I normally has a high 5-year survival rate.

The histologic subtype of the tumor, the existence of particular genetic abnormalities (such BRCA mutations), and the degree to which the cancer responds to treatment are other factors that impact prognosis.

Remember that patients with ovarian cancer continue to have better results because to improvements in medical research and individualized treatment options. It's critical to speak with medical specialists if you or someone you know is coping with ovarian cancer in order to receive accurate and current information customized to your unique circumstances.

Options for Treatment

Surgery, chemotherapy, and occasionally targeted medicines are used in the treatment of ovarian cancer. The particular strategy relies on a number of variables, including the patient's general health, the type of ovarian cancer, and the cancer's stage. An outline of popular treatment choices is provided below:

Surgery:

Debulking Surgery: Removing the tumor surgically is the main course of treatment in most cases. The goal of debulking surgery is to remove the tumor as much as feasible. A hysterectomy, or the removal of the uterus, along with the removal of the fallopian tubes and ovaries, may be required in certain situations.

Dissection of Lymph Nodes: To look for signs of cancer spread, lymph nodes in the pelvic and abdominal regions may be removed.

Chemotherapy:

Chemotherapy is frequently advised following surgery to eradicate any cancer cells that may have remained and lower the chance of recurrence.

In chemotherapy, carboplatin and paclitaxel are frequently used medications for ovarian cancer.

Specialized Treatments:

Targeted medicines that target particular molecular pathways can be effective in treating some ovarian tumors. For example, when there are particular genetic alterations, such BRCA mutations, PARP inhibitors (like olaparib and niraparib) are employed.

A monoclonal antibody called bevacizumab can be used to stop the development of blood vessels that provide cancer cells nourishment.

Immunotherapy:

A new field of study for ovarian cancer is immunotherapy, which tries to activate the immune system to identify and combat cancer cells.

Hormone Treatment:

Although hormone therapy is not frequently used to treat ovarian cancer, it might be in some circumstances, particularly when treating uncommon kinds of hormone-sensitive ovarian cancers.

Clinical Examinations:

Enrolling in clinical trials advances research on ovarian cancer and provides access to cutting-edge treatments.

Individualized treatment regimens are developed based on the unique features of the malignancy as well as the health of the patient. In order to make decisions that are appropriate for their circumstances, patients should talk through their alternatives with their healthcare team. To keep an eye out for any indications of a recurrence or treatment side effects, routine follow-up care is crucial.

Managing Breast Cancer

An ovarian cancer diagnosis can be physically and emotionally taxing for the sufferer as well as their loved ones. Coping mechanisms can guide you through this challenging process. Here are some recommendations:

Become Informed: Being aware of your diagnosis, available treatments, and what to anticipate can help you feel more in control.

Request trustworthy resources or support groups from your medical staff.

Establish a Support Network:

Family and friends: Talk to the people you care about about how you're feeling. They can offer both useful assistance and emotional support.

Support Groups: You can make connections with people going through comparable struggles by joining a support group. Talking about your experiences can be reassuring and insightful.

Seek Expert Assistance:

Counseling or Therapy: Speak with a mental health specialist who has knowledge of cancer treatment. They can guide you through coping mechanisms and feelings.

Supportive Care Services: A lot of cancer facilities provide integrative therapies, nutrition counseling, and other forms of supportive care.

Maintain Your Physical Well-Being:

Healthy Lifestyle: Pay attention to eating a balanced diet, getting adequate sleep, and continuing to be physically active (as advised by your healthcare staff).

Handle Symptoms: Coordinate closely with your medical team to handle any side effects or symptoms that may arise from your treatment.

Use Creativity to Express Yourself:

Writing in a journal, creating art, or making music can all be soothing. Think about keeping a journal, doing art, or enjoying some calming music.

Establish sensible objectives:

Daily Objectives: Divide work into doable chunks and concentrate on what you can do every day.

Celebrate Little Victories: Give thanks and recognition to little victories that you reach during your healing process.

Body-Mind Techniques:

Yoga and meditation are two mindfulness techniques that can ease stress and encourage serenity.

CHAPTER THREE

Breathing Techniques: Easy breathing techniques can help reduce anxiety and encourage calmness.

Keep Up to Date yet Avoid Information Overload:

Keep Up: Remain informed about the status of your therapy and regimen.

Limit Your Online Searches: Although it's vital to be knowledgeable, try not to overdo your research online, since this could lead to unneeded worry.

Recall that asking for assistance is acceptable and that doing so shows strength. Since each person's experience with ovarian cancer is different, choose coping mechanisms that work for you. When it comes to your emotional health, don't be afraid to be honest with your medical team. They can help you find more options and assistance.

Preventive and Prompt Identification

The management of ovarian cancer heavily relies on prevention and early detection. Although ovarian cancer cannot be completely prevented, there are some tactics that can lower the risk and improve the likelihood of early detection:

Avoidance:

Birth control pills, or oral contraceptives:

There is a link between long-term oral contraceptive use and a lower risk of ovarian cancer. Talk about this with your doctor to see whether this is a good option for you.

Being pregnant and nursing:

Pregnant and breastfeeding women may be less likely to get ovarian cancer. But each person's risk is different, and this is only one element.

Hysterectomy and tubal ligation:

Ovarian cancer risk may be decreased by surgical treatments such as hysterectomy (removal of the uterus) and tubal ligation (blocking or closing of the fallopian tubes). Individual health considerations should, however, be the basis for these judgments.

Choosing a Healthier Lifestyle:

eating a diet high in fruits and vegetables and well-balanced.

taking part in regular exercise.

staying away from tobacco products.

Genetic Testing and Counseling:

People who have a family history of breast or ovarian cancer, particularly those who have mutations in the BRCA gene, ought to think about genetic testing and counseling. Understanding your genetic risk can help with screening and preventative.

Early Identification:

Ultrasounds transvaginally and pelvic exams:

Abnormalities in the pelvic region can be found with the aid of routine transvaginal ultrasounds and pelvic exams. It's crucial to remember that these techniques are not very good in identifying ovarian cancer in its early stages.

Blood Test CA-125:

A blood test called CA-125 detects a protein that is frequently increased in ovarian cancer. Changes in CA-125 levels may be tracked in some high-risk patients or during follow-up care, despite the fact that it's not an ideal screening tool.

Awareness of Symptoms:

Recognize the possible signs of ovarian cancer, which include bloating in the abdomen, discomfort in the pelvis or abdomen, trouble eating, and changes in urination patterns. See your healthcare professional if your symptoms don't go away.

Reduced Risk Surgery:

Following pregnancy, risk-reducing procedures like salpingo-oophorectomy (removal of the ovaries and fallopian tubes) may be explored for women at high risk due to hereditary factors.

Ovarian cancer sometimes exhibits nebulous symptoms, making early detection difficult. Additionally, there is currently no standard screening test available for the general public. See your doctor for individualized guidance and necessary screening procedures if you have questions about your risk or if you have ongoing symptoms. Maintaining open lines of contact with your medical team and scheduling routine checkups are essential to the early detection and treatment of ovarian cancer.

Resilience and Continued Care

Managing life following ovarian cancer therapy requires a strong sense of survivability and follow-up care. The following are important factors for survivorship:

Rescheduled Appointments:

Keep up with your oncologist's follow-up appointments so that you can address any symptoms or concerns and have your health monitored.

While the frequency of follow-up visits may eventually decline, continuous observation is crucial for the early identification of any recurrence or any side effects of treatment.

Imaging and Examinations:

Your healthcare team may suggest routine imaging tests (such CT scans) or blood tests to check for any indications of cancer recurrence, depending on your particular circumstances.

Handling Symptoms:

Be upfront and honest with your medical staff about any new or recurring problems. Early symptom management can increase survivability and quality of life.

Psychological and Emotional Assistance:

Resilience frequently elicits a range of feelings. To address any emotional or psychological issues, think about joining a support group or going to counseling.

Mental health specialists can offer advice on coping mechanisms and emotional stability if necessary.

A Well-Being Lifestyle

Maintain a healthy lifestyle by eating a balanced diet, getting frequent exercise, and getting enough sleep.

Steer clear of smoke and drink in moderation.

Changes in Hormones and Fertility:

Talk with your healthcare team about family planning alternatives and potential issues related to fertility if fertility preservation procedures were not done prior to treatment.

Recognize and control any menopausal symptoms or hormonal changes that may occur as a result of treatment.

Effects of Treatment Over Time:

Be mindful of any possible side effects from the medication, such as weariness, neuropathy, or alterations in bone density. Talk about these with your medical team so you can successfully manage and treat them.

Genetic Testing and Counseling:

If you haven't had genetic testing and counseling, you should talk to your medical team about it. Knowing your genetic risk can help you get the treatment and screening you need throughout time.

Services for Cancer Rehabilitation:

To address any functional or mobility issues, consider seeking out rehabilitation treatments like physical therapy or occupational therapy if necessary.

After Cancer Life:

Together with your medical team, think about developing a survivorship care plan that outlines the details of your treatment and aftercare. You can use this plan as a reference for continued health management.

Being a survivor is an individual and distinct journey. Maintaining regular contact with your healthcare team, staying up to date on your health, and actively participating in your well-being management are all crucial. Frequent follow-up care gives you the chance to address any issues as soon as they arise and guarantees a thorough approach to your continued health.

CONCLUSION

Ovarian cancer is an intricate and difficult condition that necessitates a multifaceted approach to survivability, treatment, and diagnosis. Because symptoms are frequently ambiguous and there are no regular screening procedures, early detection is still a major difficulty. Research developments, individualized treatment plans, and raising awareness, however, all help to improve the prognosis for individuals impacted.

Preventive measures are essential for lowering the risk of ovarian cancer. These include genetic counseling, lifestyle modifications, and early intervention. Survivorship and follow-up care, which concentrate on keeping an eye on health, managing any long-term effects, and attending to the psychological and emotional aspects of life following treatment, are also essential parts of the trip.

It's critical for people to stay informed, actively interact with healthcare providers, and reach out to loved ones and support networks as ovarian cancer research and treatment continue to progress. The continuous progress in the fight against ovarian cancer is attributed to novel medicines, ongoing research, and a comprehensive approach to care.

In the end, ovarian cancer requires resiliency, optimism, and cooperation between patients, family members, and medical professionals. Even if there are still obstacles, everyone's dedication to early detection, prevention, awareness, and survivability creates a road towards better results and a more optimistic future for individuals who are impacted by ovarian cancer.

THE END